PRO
(e v e r y)
LIFE

Mike Novotny

Published by Straight Talk Books
P.O. Box 301, Milwaukee, WI 53201
800.661.3311 · timeofgrace.org

Printed in the United States of America
ISBN: 978-1-949488-44-9

Contents

Preface

As a pastor, I often wonder what people are thinking when I'm talking.

When I'm standing in front of church trying to remember the next point in my outline and, simultaneously, trying to personally connect with those gathered before me (or those on the other side of the camera lens), this thought races through my mind—*What are they thinking?*

Are they absorbed, or are they bored, quietly praying that the message keeps going or silently begging for a merciful *Amen*? Are they confused or enlightened, having lost my train of thought a few sentences ago or having followed the thought to new truths about God, his Son, and their salvation? Are they convicted or comforted, realizing that their lives haven't lined up with God's will or rejoicing in the good news of Jesus' love for the worst of sinners?

What exactly are all these people thinking?

Sometimes, however, I get an answer. Or lots of answers to that question. Soon after church is over, I check my in-box and read the subject lines: "Today's message . . ." "Thank you." "A few thoughts . . ." Then I open my text messages and see the various names of people who have something they want to share about the words they just heard.

Despite the initial wave of anxiety (preaching leaves me rather emotionally fragile, to be honest), I have come to appreciate those messages, whether they're filled with blush-worthy compliments or caps-lock critiques. God willing, it won't be the last time I teach on a certain topic, so knowing where people are at and how they react is a treasure to me.

Maybe it would be to you too.

Recently, I preached a three-part series on abortion, which turned out to be one of the most challenging subjects I have ever addressed in church. After each week's message, I went back to my office to find more than a few people willing to tell me what they were thinking while I was talking.

That is what I would like to share with you.

To begin I'll let you read a few emails that people sent me even before the series began, hopeful that their words would shape my words as I taught the Word. You might agree with the authors' thoughts or object to them, but I want you to hear where various people are coming from on this issue. Next I'll include the sermons themselves as I preached them so you can see what people were hearing and reacting to. Then I'll share anonymously some of the feedback I received (permission has been given, in all cases). From the woman who wished she had experienced the church's support before her teenage abortion to the stunning story about a pregnancy that was supposed to end but didn't. Next I'll offer a few comments in response to the feedback I received (I'll try to avoid being defensive or proud, I promise). Finally I'll give you some space to think, dig more deeply into God's Word, and pray.

No matter what your personal experiences with abortion, I hope this journey helps you think humbly and biblically about every womb, every woman, our world, and God's Word.

Introduction

One issue that I have intentionally not talked about is abortion. In 13 years of being a preacher, I haven't preached a single sermon on abortion. In fact, I have rarely mentioned the subject, even as a passing comment. It's not because I don't think abortion happens or that it doesn't happen often or that it hasn't happened to you. And it's not because I don't care about abortion or don't think terminating a pregnancy matters all that much. The reason I've been so hesitant is because I believe that some issues are so complex that they take time to teach well.

Teaching abortion *well* takes more than a Tweet. I've come to that conclusion, in part, because I have listened to you—your stories, your confessions, your social media posts, your responses to the surveys I've sent. And the community God has called me to serve—my church community, the community where my church is located, and our online church—thinks a lot of things about abortion. Different things. Contrasting things.

Some of you say abortion is an open-and-shut issue: "It's a baby. End of story." For others of you, however, it's not a baby but a zygote or an embryo or a fetus, a part of a woman's body that belongs to her and not to any court or church council. Some of you read the black words on the Bible's white pages—"You shall not murder"—and declare, "That settles it!" Others of you see complicated stories of rape, incest, abusive boyfriends, addicted mothers, severe genetic issues, severe mental illness, and unsupportive families; and the biblical values of compassion, kindness, and wisdom push you to see abortion as a wise and merciful option.

Some of you have never had, or even been tempted to have, an abortion. Others of you have been there. You remember the day, the weather, the room, the procedure. Some of you feel intense regret about your abortion. Others of you feel it was the best choice at the time, given the complicating factors you were facing.

Some of you try to represent Jesus by holding graphic antiabortion signs on major street corners. Others of you think it's wrong to assume that's what Jesus would do. Some of you have voted one way your entire lives simply because of abortion. Others of you believe abortion isn't the only issue a Christian should consider during an election. Some of you think pro-life means doing anything possible to protect a baby in the womb. Others of you think that "pro-life people" care more about wombs than women, a double standard that strikes you as glaringly hypocritical.

Some of you believe abortion is too controversial and political to bring up in a place like church. Others of you believe that when over 60,000,000 lives have been ended since *Roe v. Wade*, God demands that the churches say something. Some of you wish this book was on a different topic. Others of you will be hanging on every word I write.

All of that is why I've waited for some quantity time to talk about abortion. But the time has come. As long as there are unplanned pregnancies in our churches and in our world, abortion, legal or illegal, will be our issue. It will be you or your sister, your daughter or your granddaughter, your girlfriend or your wife, your roommate or your best friend. In a perfect world, every pregnancy would be wanted and planned, but this is not a perfect world. Which means abortion, at the very least, will be a temptation many of us face. So if you're ready to cover this topic, I am too.

My plan is to write about abortion in the fairest way I

know how. After reading books from both pro-life advocates and abortion doctors, surveying over 150 Christians about their experiences with abortion, studying 45 stories of women who have had abortions (and are proud of their choices), and meditating on various Bible passages that speak about this issue, I hope to communicate fairly and biblically. No straw-man arguments here or worst-case assumptions about the motives from "the other side."

My goal is to help you grasp why certain people feel one way and other people feel another, both on the morality and legality of abortion. Most important, I want to bring you back to God's Word, the place where you and I find truth to guide our lives and grace to forgive all our sins.

So before we dive into the messages I preached, let's hear from a few people who had an initial reaction to the topic itself. What did they want me to know before I opened my mouth to speak? What experiences would help me better understand what was at stake when the church talks about abortion?

Messages Received
Before the Series Began

A mother from our church shared:

> I look back through my life at my relationship with my children and think about what my response to them would be if they came to me with the simple news of expecting a child. Perhaps because I went through it myself, I know exactly how I would respond. I would respond with love and prayers and honesty and conviction. We would discuss the difficulties to come, the blessings that are promised, and the forgiveness Jesus won.
>
> So now I look back on my decision to abort and feel so sad

that [my mother], who proved her love at every opportunity and proved her faith with almost every word, did
not get the chance to share that with me. I robbed her of
the opportunity to help me. I robbed myself of the support
she would almost certainly have given me because I was
scared she would be disappointed. I was scared that she
would see what I thought of myself, that I was only worth
certain things to boys in a relationship, that my faith was
small, and that I was easily led astray. Knowing my mom,
she would have helped me live with my consequence and
helped me with whatever choice I made, adoption or
raising the child. . . . And she would have asked me how
I was feeling and if I really believed I was forgiven. She
would have talked to me about what I knew about God
and what he knows about me. And she would have encouraged me to use my experience to help others.

And yet every year, I think about that murder. I relive
it. I am horrified I could allow that to be a choice. And I
feel very low. And it doesn't get easier as the years go by.
In fact, it gets worse. I thought perhaps I would be de-
nied children later in life because of my sin, but we have
healthy children. . . . It's so easy to let the devil get a foot-
hold in these dark memories and rip my worth to shreds.
He makes me question my identity as a child of God. It's
so easy to think that I can't be forgiven. I am so grateful for groups that I can be completely transparent with
and that remind me every day how far this sin has been
removed from me because of Christ and that no matter
how hard I try to hold on to it, God's got it covered. Pray
for me tomorrow. I feel it could be a very difficult day. But
I pray that while it is good for me to feel the weight and
sorrow of my sin, the joy and peace of forgiveness is so
opposite. I will feel that eventually.

My response:

I felt so many emotions as I read this dear sister in Christ's message. Grateful for her honesty. Empathetic for the fear she felt and still sometimes feels. Humbled by her perspective. Happy that she knows the grace and forgiveness of Jesus. Relieved that she has people in her life to be "completely transparent with," people who know that the cross of Christ is the best place to take a troubled soul.

I was also taken by how ashamed she was to tell her mother about the pregnancy despite her mother's wonderfully Christ-like character. The author describes her mom as a woman who "proved her love at every opportunity" and "proved her faith with almost every word," a parent who appeared to share the grace and forgiveness of Jesus often, and yet fear stopped that conversation from happening.

I get that. I get what it's like to be surrounded by good, godly people and still feel afraid. I get what it's like to do something I regret, something embarrassing, and want to cover it up and move on. If I have felt that emotion over choices that have very little earthly impact, imagine what many women feel when giving birth could mean a completely changed life! My compassion grows the more I hear and read stories like this. What pressure people face when the pregnancy test comes back positive! What lies the father of lies must whisper in their ears to convince them to take care of things quietly!

Finally, I sensed how hard it can be for any of us to know and feel forgiven. This woman is wonderfully passionate about the Word of God, and it is rare for a Sunday to go by when I don't see her in church. I know that she spends daily time with Jesus, loves music about Jesus, and is surrounded by Jesus-loving believers. Thus, her continual battle against sorrow and shame is vivid proof that the devil is so good at accusing us and that the gospel is the daily medicine that all our souls need.

If nothing else, her email reminded me how important it would be to fill each sermon with both truth and love. Given the sensitivity of consciences like hers, perhaps love would need to get the last word.

Seeking feedback on my upcoming sermon, I sent the written draft to a few trusted friends. A coworker responded:

I am hesitant to bring this up, as I don't like the idea of wordsmithing your beautiful and heartfelt work. . . . I've got a special place in my heart for ladies who've had an abortion. My guess is I know two to four. Two for sure. I can see your point in this statement, "You can't undo the sin. Maybe now you know that you haven't just dishonored your parents or told a lie. Maybe you've murdered a child God created." Your point is valid, Mike, because abortion can't be undone like when I ask my mom to forgive me and she says yes. But I fear the statement also makes one sin worse than another or one sinner worse than another, something that I think we should be on guard about. Alternatively, perhaps one could say something along the lines of, "Look, when you were 14, you spread a rumor about the new girl at school. Look, when you were 23 and you stole that street sign with your family name on it. And if, when you were 25, you had an abortion and murdered a child God created, you committed a sin that you can't undo in the eyes of God. All three of you are in the same situation; your sin cannot be undone by your effort; your regret can't overcome your guilt." Then on to the gospel.

My response:

Aren't gospel-loving people the best? I really loved reading this brother's words because I realized that I was about to be misunderstood. My intention with the snippet that he quoted was to talk about how unfixable an abortion is—If I push you down, I can help you up. If I steal your phone, I can give it back. If I break it, I can buy it. But if I abort a child, I can't go back.

But that's not what my friend understood. He saw a subtle way that the enemy could make one sin seem worse than another, a lie that can infect the church in all kinds of ugly ways. Thus, you might soon notice when you read the sermon transcripts that follow, that the words he quoted are no longer in my message. I wanted (and needed!) to avoid the assumption that some people are better/worse than other people in the church.

One quick, final thought. I think there is a massive connection between the women we know and the way that we feel. When you have never had an abortion and never known/loved a person who has had an abortion, it is all too tempting to rattle off a few Bible passages, make a simplistic conclusion about life, and move on with your day. But when, like the author of this note, you have walked with people who are facing an unplanned pregnancy, your heart often softens. The circumstances of each situation open your eyes to layers of complexity, complication, and temptation. I would encourage you, therefore, to read, talk, and listen to stories of women who have had or considered having an abortion. In my experience, that knowledge is necessary before you are equipped to speak with grace, truth, and wisdom.

A woman whom I know who, by God's grace, has worked through some tremendous trauma, emailed me days before the series began:

Abortion is a hard topic that most churches never cover, and I appreciate that you are. It is very sensitive to a lot of people, but I simply cannot stop thinking that I hope that you cover the idea that not everyone who has had an abortion chose it of their own free will. That is NEVER spoken of, ever. In any circle. Not even among counselors. I have known multiple other people who have been through it, even had another classmate go through it as a child. Which makes me sad and feel old, like I have way too many stories. But when you do share, so many women say, me too. It's real, and yet no one addresses it. It's so much harder to deal with in the Christian church. Abortion is a sin, so what we did is a sin. That pain then becomes shame and something to hide. This horrific thing is accidentally blamed on the victim all the time because no one thinks to say, "But not in this situation," because no one wants to admit it happens. I just wanted to bring that up because so many women will be listening to Time of Grace, *and some of them will have been through that. They may never have told anyone yet bear the deep scars of losing a child to something they did not choose, a child that society tells them they should want to get rid of anyway because it was conceived in abuse. Yet it hurt them to have it taken from them. Then they are called sinners for going through it. It's crazy hard. I am so blessed to have my husband by my side who helped me walk through that and allowed me to grieve as I needed to. With his help I am doing well.*

My response:

Wow . . . where would my heart even start to respond? As a father of two daughters, this story saddens me to an inexpressible degree. I cannot fathom what our Father must feel when his beloved daughters are treated this way.

When a woman is abused, assaulted, impregnated, forced to abort, and then blamed and labeled by Christians who claim to stand with God on the side of what's good? I shudder at the thought.

Looking back on the sermon series, this woman's point is one I wish I had addressed better. My messages ended up being some of the longest that I have ever preached (the first one ended at 52 minutes, 50 percent longer than my average), so it grieves me to say that I didn't spend much time addressing forced abortions connected to assault/incest. While statistically they make up a small percentage of all abortions (Planned Parenthood suggests less than .5 percent), this woman's story is a reminder how real and relevant the issue still is. And, as she points out, she is not alone.

My regret in rereading the transcripts of my sermons is not having said more during the messages themselves. Honestly, I intended to but lost track of this goal during the rush of preparation. However, I pray that God helps abuse victims read these words and know the truth: It is not your fault.

I will write that again—It is not your fault.

Since an abuse expert reminded me that I can never say those words too much, I'll repeat—It is not your fault.

Years ago I read a book about sexual assault in which the author made a wise distinction between the shame we feel for sins we commit and the shame we feel for sins committed against us. It can be hard for some Christians to remember that sometimes sex and abortion are not rebellious acts of the sinful will but horrific tragedies forced on innocent victims.

If you or someone you love has been abused, I hope you can find the three messages I preached on the issue of abuse. In particular, I spent the entire first message speaking to people who have been victimized, offering them hope and healing through Jesus. Please find those messages online (go to timeofgrace.org and search for the series *Abuse: What Does God Say?*). God willing, like this woman's husband, those words will be your guide to the loving arms of God.

This final note I want to share with you is lengthy, but I found it extremely helpful in grasping so many of the dynamics a woman might feel in her spiritual journey before, during, and after an abortion, so I'll let you read her words in their entirety:

I know that Pastor Novotny will be preaching on abortion the week after next at The CORE. It's one of the things that is compelling me to share this now.

I sat in a chair in his congregation last Sunday—visiting from out of state—and was too ashamed to talk to him after the worship service. Too ashamed to ask to take Communion. Afraid he might recognize my face from a social media message and recognize that it was me, the one who shared that I had had an abortion—even though I know with the thousands of followers, he probably would not. Even though it shouldn't matter if he did. I've been working on "healing" for just about a year now from abortion and still couldn't bring myself to face one of the few pastors out there who I thought might actually "get it."

I feel compelled to share this . . . this article? My story? I don't know what to call it. I want people to understand that there are people like me, people who are just living in overwhelming shame, sitting next to them, sitting in the pew in their congregations. I want the other women like me to know they are not alone. I want people to understand the thought process that kept me from surrendering my secret to anyone, especially the church. And yet, I'm still dealing with the shame and afraid to share.

It'll be obvious that I'm not a professional writer. I don't have it all done with footnotes with references, but I'm sure you will recognize the Bible verses referenced, and I can get research statistics. It's something I wrote as I couldn't sleep. I'm supposed to be writing my testimony, yet stuff like this comes out instead. It might give Pastor Mike one more perspective that he may not have heard as he finishes writing his sermon on abortion. I'm finding my perspective is slightly different than other women who have shared their abortion stories with me this past year—women who had their abortions before becoming a Christian, but similar to those who were Christians at the time of it.

I sat in the pew for 26 years, suffering overwhelming guilt and shame and unwilling to surrender my secret, confess my sin. Thirty years ago, I found myself pregnant out of wedlock. At first, I was ecstatic. The only thing I had ever wanted my entire life was to be a wife and mother. I was missing the wife part, but I was thrilled nonetheless . . . until I shared that news with the only real support network I had: my mom, who was the sweetest, most God-fearing Christian I knew. She told me to get an abortion.

I was shocked. I was devastated.

The only other people I shared the news of my pregnancy with, two of my sisters, agreed with my mom. When I protested that it was against God's will, one of them cited a Bible passage that God formed Adam, then breathed life into him, drawing the parallel to a baby being formed in the womb, then not having "life" until taking its first breath.

I was defeated. I would have no support if I proceeded with carrying this child.

Then my boss laid me off. Now, not only would I not have emotional support, but my financial means to support this child just disappeared. I wasn't aware of pregnancy resource centers. I didn't know of state welfare agencies. I had left the church—not because I didn't believe in God— but because of the hurt a person in the church caused and my lack of maturity to realize that we're all sinful, hurtful people. We're all hypocrites. Whatever the case, I didn't believe the church was an option to find help either. I believed that I deserved what I got. I deserved to face the consequences of my actions (which is absolutely true). I just wrongfully thought that the consequence that I deserved was for my child to be ripped from my womb.

So with my now ex-boss paying for the abortion and my mom driving me to the clinic, I did the most horrific, unthinkable thing . . . I consented to killing my child.

The abortion itself was reminiscent of being raped in many ways. And that sound of a vacuum . . . sucking the life right out of me. It is a sound I will never forget. I laid there sobbing. Alone. Sobbing for the life I just took, sobbing for allowing men to do whatever they wanted with my body that got me pregnant, sobbing for who I was and who I would never be.

I remember slowly climbing into the car to go home and driving past the people holding the condemning signs that reminded me of what I had done and what I now deserved . . . hell. I cried for days, weeping for the baby I would never hold in my arms because I m-u-r-d-e-r-e-d her. I cried until I had no tears left to cry. Left empty. Empty of tears. My womb now empty. Empty as my aching heart. Empty as my arms that longed to hold that baby. The baby I was responsible for murdering. I longed for my death and daydreamed about the many ways I could end it. I deserved death. And I deserved the punishment it would bring for me to live out eternity in hell.

Time marched on. But the pain didn't subside. It was always there. Time does not heal all wounds, no matter what people say. Not on its own anyways.

I eventually married a guy who really had no idea of what he was getting into with me. Besides letting him know just how bad of a sinner he would be marrying, I never again spoke of the abortion after telling him . . . until 30 years later. The shame and overwhelming guilt of what I had done lived in me. It defined me. But if I could help it, not another living soul was going to know just how sinful I was. I was determined to take that secret to the grave.

I miscarried three times during our first years of marriage. I felt it was a fitting punishment that I deserved. Reliving the horror of what I had done as I had to go through a D&C (note: a D&C is one method of abortion) seemed very fitting. I deserved it. I deserved God taking away these children after I destroyed my first child so carelessly. Then my fifth pregnancy. It completely changed my life. I spent the first 12 weeks on bedrest, and once I hit that 12-week mark, I had my first inkling of hope. Hope that God would allow me the blessing of actually holding one of my babies.

At 24 weeks into my pregnancy, I started having some pain. I called my doctor and was told to come in immediately. My worst fear confirmed. I was in preterm labor. Back to bedrest. I was so worried that I was once again going to lose one of my precious children. I didn't deserve a child, and I was very well aware of that fact. But I wanted that baby with every fiber of my being. I prayed like I had never prayed before. I bargained with God. Making him promises that I would not let my child make the same mistakes I did, that I would bring her up in the training and admonition of the Lord in a home where his Word was lived out. That I would read the Bible regularly, take her to church. I would protect her and keep her as safe as humanly possible.

God answered my prayers. And, ironically, I must have had some integrity because I took a little pride in the fact that I kept my promises—so I kept my bargain with him. My beautiful little angel—and that is exactly how I looked at her—a messenger from God, was born healthy in every way. My first mission was to get her baptized as quickly as possible. She was not promised tomorrow, and I knew that only too well.

My husband, who was out to sea when she was born, was allowed to fly off the ship and come home for a week. We contacted a couple of churches, only to be told that they would not baptize her until we took and finished Bible information classes with them. There was no time for that. My husband needed to be there for her baptism, and the government demanded he go back on the ship and be gone for several months. She was not promised a tomorrow. She needed to be baptized NOW in case the unthinkable happened to her. She needed to be made a disciple of God. Whoever is baptized will be saved. You must be born of water and the Spirit. These verses from my childhood swirled in my mind. I could not wait the nine months before my husband would return from cruise.

Finally, I contacted the church that I myself had been baptized at when I was a baby, the church I attended as a child. It was such a long shot, I thought. We had moved away almost 15 years prior when I was a child, and I did not go back there when we moved back to the area several years later. I was disgruntled with all churches and the "hypocrites" that were in them by then, and I didn't go to ANY church. But now I found myself in that very awkward position where I had to return to a church to fulfill my end of the bargain to God. To my complete surprise, the pastor said he would be happy to baptize her . . . as long as we promised to raise her up in the church. He took a gamble that we would keep that promise—I would not have been so trusting with two strangers who didn't have a church home and admitted they hadn't been to church since they were married, hadn't been to church before that for several years. But he did. That Saturday, we were able to have her baptized surrounded by our immediate family. I may have been many things, a sinful, promiscuous slut . . . a murderer, but I was one with some integrity who kept my promises.

The next Sunday was the first of a lifetime of Sundays back in worship. Although back in the pew, I really didn't think there was hope for me. "You know that no murderer has eternal life abiding in her" (1 John 3:15).

This was for my daughter, so SHE would spend eternity in heaven. So that the Holy Spirit would have the opportunity to work faith in her (faith comes from hearing the message and the message is heard through the word of Christ). Time passed, and I started wondering if maybe God's forgiveness was for me too. Those words of his I was hearing every Sunday, could they possibly be for me too?

Then I got pregnant. My sixth pregnancy. I was overjoyed with the thought of another child. A little baby brother or sister for my daughter. Another blessing from God. Was this confirmation that God did forgive me? And then, all my symptoms of pregnancy stopped . . . was I just far enough along for the morning sickness to subside? At my in-laws' house, as we transferred from one duty station to another, in another unfamiliar, uncompassionate doctor's office, I looked at the ultrasound screen and saw no heart beating on the little body on the screen. Another child I would never hold in my arms. Another D&C. Another reminder of what I had done. Another reminder that I deserved nothing, especially nothing good. Another confirmation that God's forgiveness was NOT for me.

But I continued with my promise and kept taking my

daughter to church, going to Bible study, reading the Bible to her almost every day, praying for her faith to be strong, and praying that God would somehow hear and grant my prayer for another child to hold someday. The years went by. God fulfilled my prayer for more children. However, along with the living, were more miscarriages too. I did everything I could in church and in my life to live a life that would set the example for the children God blessed me with. . . . I didn't believe this was for my benefit—a way to earn my way to heaven, because I still didn't believe that I was forgiven and that heaven was for me. I shared Jesus' forgiveness—The Great Exchange—he made with sinners. There were days, even years at a time, when I thought just maybe that included me. I joined some pro-life groups along the way. Wanting to spare others the pain and torment of what I was living with but too ashamed to share my why, to share my story of why I was involved in the pro-life movement. When I got too close to needing to explain why I was involved, I disappeared from that movement. Having to make another military move gave me the perfect excuse.

On the outside, I was the picture of a Christian wife and mother. I doubt anyone guessed at the secret I kept locked away.

A number of things happened in my life in quick succession. I became so overwhelmed dealing with those things that I sought Christian counseling. Then one day, the secret I thought I would never share with another soul came pouring forth out of my mouth. I wanted to put it back. Shove it back in the closet. But like Pandora's box, the evils of my past were now out in the open.

"Confess your sins to each other . . . so that you may be healed" (James 5:16).

With that confession came a number of things. The first, hearing God's forgiveness spoken to me through one of his servants . . . although I had heard those words repeated almost every Sunday for the last 26 years, that was the first time I heard them spoken for THAT sin, the sin I believed was unforgivable. I wanted him to tell me it, over and over again. Then the hard journey to healing began.

Unfortunately, hearing you are forgiven does not equal feeling that you are.

Healing is slow in coming. I've been told it's like an onion, that it happens in layers or like waves in the ocean. I often feel like it's one step forward and ten steps back. I still struggle daily with my identity in Christ. That there truly is no condemnation for me. That he can forgive even the unforgivable. That the Great Exchange is for even the likes of me.

As I heal, I feel God is placing on my heart the need to share what I'm learning with those others who are sitting in the pew, silently suffering. And not only them but also to share with the people sitting next to them and the people preaching to them. The church, where "we"—those who have committed the unmentionable—have the contradiction of feeling judged and condemned by everyone around us and yet it being the only place where we can get true healing.

To help the church understand that, yes, we have sinned but remind them that Jesus said, "Let him who has no sin, cast the first stone." For if the numbers are correct, there are a lot of others sitting in the pew feeling the same condemnation and guilt that I felt all those years. That I still struggle with.

I'm sharing my story because I was sitting in your church. I was one of your parishioners. I was sitting next to you in church and Bible study. I taught your children at vacation Bible school. I led your women's group. I was your prayer warrior. I was your pro-life activist. I loved and cared for you, encouraged you with God's Word, brought you meals when you were sick, babysat your kids, had you over for Sunday football games after church. For 26 years.

I didn't keep silent to try and deceive you—well maybe a little. I didn't want you to know just how much of a sinner I was. I kept silent because I'm so ashamed of my past. Because I live with the shame and guilt every day. Because I was afraid of your judgment and condemnation. Because I know that I don't deserve anything but it.

I'm sharing my story in case YOU are one of my other sisters (or brothers) in Christ, sitting in the pew, hoping no one will discover your past sins. I'm sharing my story in hopes that God may use my story to let you know that you don't have to suffer in silence anymore. That there is no condemnation in Christ Jesus now. That his forgiveness is for YOU. That the water of YOUR baptism washed you clean. That Christ's suffering on the cross was to redeem YOU.

He paid for it all. Confess your sins to one another so you can be healed.

My response:

If I've ever felt a tidal wave of emotions after reading an email, it was this one. This gracious woman shared so many details in such a transparent way with so many scriptural truths that I struggled to find the words to respond to her email.

I once heard someone say that when you read a book, you are absorbing ten years of hard-won wisdom from the author's life. This email had that effect on me. In one email, I felt like I had learned a thousand things I never knew before, lessons that I would carry with me into my first message on abortion, which is why this woman's story would appear not once but twice in my opening message on the topic of abortion.

While I am tempted to type 79 things I feel when reading her words, let me narrow down my reaction to two points—"We/They" and gospel dominance.

First, the issue of "We/They." When you haven't committed a certain sin, it is natural to assume that other people in the room haven't either. For example, if you have never used heroin or been physically abusive or gotten hooked on pornography, you might assume that your friends or your family or your small group Bible study is all in the same boat.

We all know that such things are wrong. We would never do that. We would not be tempted by that. Maybe they, out there in the world, would do that, but not here in the church.

This woman's email reminds us to never assume anything. "I was one of your parishioners. I was sitting next to you in church and Bible study. I taught your children at vacation Bible school. I led your women's group. I was your prayer warrior. I was your pro-life activist. I loved and cared for you, encouraged you with God's Word, brought you meals when you were sick, babysat your kids, had you over for Sunday football games after church. For 26 years."

Imagine a passing comment about abortion at a Bible study she attended. Imagine the blunt comments about Planned Parenthood or "those people" when she herself was one of "those people." Imagine what such words would do to her already struggling soul.

I believe it is spiritually necessary to assume that "we" are "they." We who follow Jesus have done and said and chosen everything that "they" have out in the world. We might regret it. We might confess it. But we still do it. We still think it. We still carry the wounds. And we need the tenderness and empathy of one another.

So please remember who we are.

Second, please let the gospel dominate the places where you gather. Your home. Your church. Your emails. Your text threads. This sister's quarter-century struggle with shame is not unique. As a pastor, I see this up close all the time. Especially as we open the Bible and see how much a holy God hates sin, it is a daily battle to believe that Jesus paid for every sin. For all our sins.

For that sin.

They say that you need nine nice comments for every one critical comment. Perhaps there is a spiritual parallel, namely, that you need nine paragraphs about the forgiveness of Jesus for every paragraph about God's hatred of sin. Maybe our hearts are wired in a way to need an imbalance of sorts, a message that leans far to the side of grace and mercy.

I hope the end of my first sermon does that very thing, letting the blood of Jesus have the final word on the topic of abortion.

Before we jump into that first sermon, however, I'd love for you to pause and pour out your heart on the page.

Take a moment to examine your own heart and see what's going on there. Once you're done, we'll be ready to open our Bibles and talk about the womb, the women, and the world God has placed us in.

After reading this far, how are you feeling?

Trust in the Lord with all your heart and lean not on your own understanding; in all your ways submit to him, and he will make your paths straight.

Proverbs 3:5,6

If you had the chance to reply to the previous emails, what words would you choose?

What personal situations are you remembering?

What stories of loved ones are you recalling?

What Bible passages, if any, are coming to mind?

All Scripture is God-breathed and is useful for teaching, rebuking,
correcting and training in righteousness, so that the servant of God
may be thoroughly equipped for every good work.

2 Timothy 3:16,17

What fears are you facing?

What questions are you hoping I'll answer?

Praise the LORD, my soul; all my inmost being, praise his holy name. Praise the LORD, my soul, and forget not all his benefits—who forgives all your sins and heals all your diseases, who redeems your life from the pit and crowns you with love and compassion.

Psalm 103:1–4

Sermon 1
Abortion and the Womb

Despite their radically different views on abortion, both pro-life and pro-choice people can agree on one thing: People matter. Each individual person matters. Which is why starting our discussion with the womb is so essential. Before we can talk about the reproductive rights of people, the national legislation that affects people, and how best to help people with unplanned pregnancies, we must first ask how many people we are hoping to help.

As we zoom into the womb, is that combination of sperm and egg a part of the mother whom we care about, or is it a separate person whom we also care about? Is that a baby to care for or a clump of cells that could one day become a baby to care for? Is that a unique person with the human right to be protected from danger, or does the woman have the right to do what she desires with that unique part of her own body? The more I've read and studied and wrestled with abortion, the more convinced I am that the first thing we need to figure out with abortion is how many people are involved in the process.

I say that because we all know what to do with a person. Imagine a one-year-old standing on stage with me, someone whom we would all agree is a person worthy of our love and care. Can you picture a little girl like that, just learning to walk, with her pigtails just long enough to poke out of the top of her head? No matter your religion or political party, we would all agree that she is a person, right?

That adorable (albeit imaginary) girl is our common ground. She's a person.

The fact that she is a person would remain true even if I revealed to you that this little girl had a very complicated story. If we learned that this one-year-old wasn't planned by her father or wasn't really wanted by her mother, would any of you say that she stops being a person? Do we reclassify her as a thing, an "it" instead of a "she"? While we might lament her parents' lack of love, I think we would still consider her a person.

What if I told you her father was verbally abusive or mother was chemically dependent on heroin, that there was no guarantee that her dad would seek help for his controlling behavior or her mom would get sober anytime soon? Would those heartbreaking details move that little girl into the category of cells, bees, and trees, things instead of people? I don't think so.

What if, God forbid, I whispered to you that she was conceived through assault or through incest? Would you consider it merciful to find a doctor who could stop her heart from beating and her lungs from breathing?

What if her parents had other plans for work, for college, or for life that this one-year-old put on hold or changed entirely? We might offer a compassionate word to Mom and offer to lend a hand to Dad, but I don't think that their desires would change the little girl's status as one of us, a person worthy of life, liberty, and the pursuit of happiness.

What if the one-year-old had Down's syndrome or a genetic issue or a physical abnormality? Or what if the mother just didn't want to do the diaper and stroller and 2:00 A.M. feedings again?

My guess is that all the situations above would elevate your empathy, increase your compassion, and call you to selfless action, but they wouldn't change your answer about who that little girl is. She's still a person.

Do you see the importance of this issue? We all know what to do with people. People come from their mothers, but they are not part of their mothers. They are people. Small people, weak people, defenseless people, still developing people but still people. God says this about such people: **"Defend the weak. . . . Uphold the cause of the poor and the oppressed. Rescue the weak and the needy"** (Psalm 82:3,4).

So *the* question that shapes our view of abortion is this: Is that a person in the womb? On the first day or after the first month or during the second trimester, is that a person? While love urges me to talk to you first about all the circumstances of an unplanned pregnancy (which I will next time), logic requires me to start with the essential question—When does life begin? When do people become people?

In my research of both pro-life and pro-choice materials, I have found five answers to that question. Before I open my Bible, let's look at what those five are:

First, some say a person is created at conception. And, they would add, science proves it. Nearly every cell in a woman's body shares the same genetic code—her lungs and heart and appendix are stamped with almost entirely identical DNA. But when sperm meets egg, something new appears. The DNA is different. At a crime scene, we treasure the uniqueness of genetics, relying on the differences to help us solve cases. Could the same be true for the womb?

Or marvel at how the fingerprints on those tiny developing fingers are unique from the swirls on the tips of the mother's fingers. Or consider that unless a woman has two hearts, two lungs, four legs, and four eyes, there must be a separate person inside of her.

Perhaps such reasons are why numerous medical textbooks on biology and embryology, *TIME*, and *Rand McNally Atlas of the Body and Mind* all agree with the point the *New En-*

cyclopedia Britannica made in saying, "A new individual is created when the elements of a potent sperm merge with those of a fertile egg."[1] In other words, life begins at conception.

Second, others are convinced that people are created at recognition. Just watch what is in the womb and see if you don't recognize that as a little person. Look at that little peanut with the beating heart, little nose, and countable toes. Doesn't that look like a human? If we showed the latest ultrasound to a group of preschoolers who had never heard of abortion, what would they say? I haven't run any test trials, but I bet they would recognize that as a yet-to-be-born person.

That's what happened to Abby Johnson. Abby was the Planned Parenthood director who was asked, unexpectedly, to assist with an abortion. The doctor was using an ultrasound during the procedure, which meant Abby was able to see something she recognized. She noticed the tiny vertebrae of the little spine. She gasped as the fetus reacted to the approaching instrument. And she knew it was a person. Recognition shaped, even changed, her views about abortion.

Third, others say a person is created at viability. Viability is a fancy word that means that you have the ability to live. If you were born, you could survive. Given our modern NICU technology, infants can survive birth long before hitting 40 weeks of gestation. The current record is just around 21 weeks, a number that would have shocked 99.99 percent of humans who have ever lived on Earth. But earlier than that? Dr. Willie Parker is one of the few abortion doctors in the American South, and he makes the viability argument here: "Before 22 weeks, a fetus is not in any way equal to 'a baby' or 'a child.' . . . Every one of the fetal parts—head, body, limbs—like a puzzle that has to be put back together. . . . I place them together, re-creating the fetus in the pan. I have done this so many times that it has become routine: no matter what these parts may look like, this is organic matter that does not add up to anything that can live on its own."[2] This thing in the womb can't live. So that's not life. Not yet.

Fourth, still others say a person is created by desire. Shout *Your Abortion* is a collection of stories from women who are unashamed of their choice to abort. One of the women, Amy, makes the argument about desire when she says, "The simple truth is this: if a sperm and egg come together when a child is desired, a human being is born. But if a sperm and egg come together when a woman knows in her bones that it is not the right time for her to be a mother, then perhaps what is born is her own confident agency over her life."[3] If the time isn't right, if the desire isn't there, then a human being isn't there. That isn't a person. Not until her mother wants it to be so.

Finally, some say a person is created at birth. Personhood is obvious then. We can see that this isn't a part of the mother's body but its own unique entity. But until the moment they leave the womb, this is part of the mother, her business, under her wisdom and judgment and authority, since no one can know a woman's body better than the woman herself.

These are the top answers to the key question of personhood—at conception, at recognition, at viability, at desire, or at birth. Have you heard all of those arguments? How about you personally? If I gave you a moment to consider when you personally believe life begins and why, which option would you choose? And what would you say to people who choose the other four? And, a bigger issue, an infinitely more important issue—What does God say? If you are a Christian who calls God your Father and Jesus your Savior and the Holy Spirit your Truth-definer, which of those five options does God agree with? We can talk about the complications of unplanned pregnancy in the next sermon and the political impact, if any, the sermon after that. But for now, let's answer this: What should a Christian believe about the most important issue on abortion, the issue of personhood?

A few Bible passages help us answer that question. First, the story of jumping John and baby Jesus. In Luke chapter 1, Mary is just pregnant with Jesus, and she goes to see her relative Elizabeth, who is six months along with the soon-to-be-named John the Baptist. When Mary shows up and says hi to Elizabeth, John, in the womb, acts like someone just turned on that House of Pain song and starts to jump around. The Scripture says, **"When Elizabeth heard Mary's greeting, the baby leaped in her womb"** (verse 41). The Greek word originally used here for *baby* is *brephos*. What was in her womb was a *brephos*? Okay, but couldn't that mean fetus or something other than baby? Now jump ahead to Luke chapter 2. Mary makes it to Bethlehem, pushes out Jesus, lays him in a manger, and an angel shows up to the shepherds and says, **"This will be a sign to you: You will find a baby wrapped in cloths and lying in a manger"** (verse 12). Want to guess what Greek word is used for *baby*? *Brephos*. So in the Bible's own language, John in the womb is a *brephos* and Jesus outside of it is a *brephos*. A baby. So saying that babies don't exist until birth isn't biblical. And if Elizabeth was only six months along, with the technology of two thousand years ago and not the NICU of today, viability can't be biblical either. Two options down, three others to go.

So is it conception, recognition, or desire? Psalm 139 helps here when King David says to God, **"For you created my inmost being; you knit me together in my mother's womb. Your eyes saw my unformed body"** (verses 13,16). "My unformed body. Before my body was formed, before you could recognize the little fingers or hear the heartbeat, that was 'my' body; that was 'me.'" Me. David as a person began before he was recognizable. And notice who did it? God. God created that body. God desired to make David. Therefore, the creation of a new person doesn't begin when a mother desires a child but when our heavenly Father does.

This is God's answer to our very human desire to claim authority over what belongs to God. I noticed this theme in *Shout Your Abortion.* One woman said, "My belief is the absolute right to bodily autonomy."[4] Chrissy added, "I deserve to exist in the world as an autonomous and liberated entity."[5] Wendy, a former U.S. Senator, preached, "You are the only person who can decide what is right for you."[6] Where many people disagree with God is not just with the womb but with their entire selves. But Christians believe that God made us. He gave us life. We are not our own. We were made and saved, not to be lord and master but to follow the Lord who gave his life for us.

That leaves us with one option—conception. Which is exactly what Psalm 51:5 proves: **"Surely I was sinful at birth, sinful from the time my mother conceived me."** Here David admits how far back his sin problem went, stretching all the way back to his conception. But *things* aren't sinful. A tree or a chair or a clump of cells isn't good or evil, moral or immoral, godly or sinful. So if David says that he was sinful from his conception, he is saying that his conception created . . . a person.

The saying we sometimes hear, then, is scriptural: *Life begins at CONCEPTION.* Yes, there is lots of developing to do. Yes, that child still needs its mother to survive those first weeks. Yes, we hope every child is a desired child. But our Father has gone on the record in Old Testament and New to tell us that life begins at conception. An abortion, therefore, doesn't scrape off some cells. An abortion ends a life. A choice not to abort, therefore, saves a life that God loves.

I know you probably have a ton of questions. But what if you're not ready to be a father or if you don't have money to raise a daughter or if you're already depressed or don't want to be bound forever to an abusive man? What will the church do when someone gets pregnant and didn't plan to? How will we love all the lives involved—baby and mother and father? How can you and I move past the shallow love that just votes and then stops and dive deep into sacrificial love for complicated families? And how does all this affect our politics and policies and sense of justice? That's what's coming up in the next two sermons, so I hope you keep reading.

But there's one thing I still need to say. Something she needed me to tell you. Last week I got the longest email I've gotten in a long time from a woman who gave me permission to tell you about her abortion. She didn't want one, honestly, until her mother, the most God-fearing woman she knew, told her to get one. And then her sisters reasoned that it wasn't a person until its first breath, until birth. So feeling completely alone, she agreed. And for years afterward, decades actually, she struggled to believe that she could be forgiven.

Maybe you feel that way too. Maybe long ago or just this week you ended a pregnancy. Maybe you're the guy who pushed it, who paid for it, or who didn't say anything and just let her do it. Maybe you're the mom or the dad who was embarrassed, the Christian family that didn't want the pregnancy to prove you weren't that perfect after all. Maybe you had some good reasons. Maybe not. But maybe now, with an open Bible, you realize what happened. That a life was ended.

If so, read this: Jesus Christ, the *brephos* born in Bethlehem, came into this world to forgive and save people just like you. Jesus was nicknamed the Son of David, his ancient ancestor, and he wasn't ashamed of the name even though David once committed . . . murder. And when Jesus took his friends up to a mountaintop and showed them his glory, who appeared at his side? Elijah and Moses, who happened to be . . . a murderer. And when Jesus wanted the good news of his forgiveness for all sinners to go beyond Israel, to whom did he appear? To Saul (aka Paul), a man with a history of murder. The fact that God chose this same Moses, this very David, this Paul to write most of the Bible, despite their pasts, should tell you that Jesus saves us from the worst of it. That through Jesus, you too can be saved.

Listen to Jesus' friend John: **"If we confess our sins, he is faithful and just and will forgive us our sins and purify us from all unrighteousness"** (1 John 1:9). Jesus is faithful. Jesus will forgive our sins. Jesus will purify us. From what? From *all* unrighteousness. From all of it! The reason Jesus was conceived of the Holy Spirit and born of the virgin Mary was so that he could suffer under Pontius Pilate, die, and be buried. Why? So that he could rise on the third day and proclaim forgiveness of sins to Paul, to me, to you. Remember Abby from Planned Parenthood? That day with the ultrasound changed her life, but it couldn't undo her support of abortion or her own two abortions. So she ran to Jesus. And now she says, "Good Friday has never been the same for me since."[7]

The woman who emailed me agrees. She concluded her incredible email with these words: "I'm sharing my story in case YOU are one of my other sisters (or brothers) in Christ, sitting in the pew, hoping no one will discover your past sins. I'm sharing my story in hopes that God may use my story to let you know that you don't have to suffer in silence anymore. That there is no condemnation in Christ Jesus now. That his forgiveness is for YOU. That the water of YOUR baptism washed you clean. That Christ's suffering on the cross was to redeem YOU. He paid for it all. Confess your sins to one another, so you can be healed."

Friends, there is life in the womb. And there is eternal life in the One from heaven.

Viewer Reactions to "Abortion and the Womb"

An online listener immediately responded:

Thank you for delving into the controversial topic of abortion. It is definitely not one covered in the church often but one that urgently needs Scripture's interpretation. It's a topic very dear to me (not from experience but just a personal passion—my master's degree thesis was on the topic. I've done volunteer work at a pregnancy and life center, and we regularly donate to pro-life organizations). If you're receiving any negative feedback from the topic, just know you're doing the right thing by talking so in depth about the subject.

My response:

You're welcome. I am receiving some negative feedback on the topic, so I appreciate your encouragement to keep speaking in depth. I would ask for your prayers since "talking in depth" and "talking with wisdom" can be two different things. My personality finds it natural to dive deeply into topics, but speaking with wisdom, empathy, and balance are often a struggle for me, so please ask the Spirit to help me say the right thing at the right time to the right people.

A Christian man from our church emailed:

I am speechless and commend you for every word. GOD used you to bring one of the most powerful sermons I have ever heard. Amen.

My response:

Thank you for the kind words. Even more, thank you for the caps-lock GOD. Only a GOD who is infinitely good, gracious, forgiving, kind, compassionate, and faithful is able to change people's minds, erase people's guilt, and stir people's desire to love others. My words lack such power, but GOD is able!

A newer member of our congregation told me after church that she wanted to email me some thoughts. Soon after, she wrote:

Let me just say again what an informative, gripping, and powerful message! This sermon series has gripped me and brought me to the edge of my seat wanting more!

There has never been any doubt in my mind that conception is the start of life. I rejoiced and cherished every minute of my pregnancies. New life was growing inside me. God had blessed us three times over!

Though I cherished and rejoiced with the news of each pregnancy, I know that this is not the case for all who find themselves expecting a child. There is incest, rape, abuse, addiction, financial struggles, not ready, illness, and the list goes on. Though, to me, these are still not causes for termination of life. There are those who do not believe that life starts at conception. They don't know Jesus. They don't have faith.

In the event of an unbeliever finding themselves with an unwanted pregnancy, and after counseling, I have been

there for three women who moved forward with termina-
tion. I know, with my beliefs, what they were doing went
against every fiber of my being. It was with these three
women that I showed the love of Jesus by offering love,
grace, and compassion. I walked with them, kept their se-
crets, and offered support before and after. It was much
later that these women came to know Jesus. It was at this
time that I was able to tell of love, grace, compassion, and
forgiveness of sins. They don't need to continue to feel the
guilt and shame of the choice that was made.

I am pro-life; however, not everyone has the same
Christian beliefs. We still need caring and trained profes-
sionals to help these women through what could be the
darkest time of their lives. We need safe environments
for these terminations to take place; and when the time
comes, if it be the day, weeks, months, or years after, we
need to be there to show them the way to forgiveness
from guilt and shame.

Looking forward to the next part of this sermon topic.

My response:

I cannot tell you how much I love people like this
woman. John, one of Jesus' closest friends, once
wrote that our Savior is **"full of grace and truth"**
(John 1:14). In the same way, our Father wants all his
children to be the same—never being "half-truth"
or "some grace" but being full of both.

As this sister in Christ and I dialogued together,
we talked about how to love someone who is going
through with an abortion. What do you do? What do
you say? To what extent do you offer support? How
can we maximize love without ever compromising

the truth? How can we ask God to bless someone without blessing everything that someone does?

There are no simple answers to these questions, but this committed sister in Christ is a wonderful example of someone who refuses to sit on the sidelines and criticize but instead jumps into the deep end of messy situations in order to bring as much Jesus as she can to people in need.

Another member of our church emailed me a few days after this first message:

I just wanted to thank you for the fantastic teaching in the first abortion segment. So clear and thorough and scriptural and logical and emotional. Perfect truth—lots of truth—and grace. . . . I know two women who have had abortions (that I know of). Both were during college in the 1980s, both Christians worried about what people would think. Both lived to regret it, and it took years for each of them to feel forgiven.

I know another woman who became pregnant years ago while in college in the '90s at age 20. It was a one-night stand after drinking too much. She had been loosely raised Catholic but had lived in an abusive household. Away at college, finding herself pregnant without a healthy support system, her mother gave her the money to drive to Madison (the only place in Wisconsin at that time where an abortion was available) and take care of the "problem." She has told me that she was on the table, draped, and moments away from the procedure when she decided she couldn't do it. She had known in her heart that it was wrong but had just been carried along with what seemed like the right solution under the circumstances.

Abandoning the procedure that far along in the process is almost unheard of. This woman is the birth mother of one of our adopted sons. I have known her since her fifth month of pregnancy and was with her to support her during childbirth. She has said repeatedly from that day and through the years that her decision to bear this child and place him with us for adoption makes her so happy and was the best thing she's ever done. We praise God for our son. (This is a whole amazing story, full of details God had clearly planned, that we watched unfold before our very eyes!)

Another interesting item along the theme of "desire" for a child: I don't know if you remember Jocelyn Elders, the US Health & Human Services Secretary during the Clinton era. One of her mantras was, "Every child should be a planned and wanted child." (I can still hear her voice proclaiming this.) She promoted federal funding and expansion of abortion so that no unplanned or unwanted child needed to cause suffering, or suffer, by being born. Somewhere during those years, I realized that our whole family would not exist if this was the case. I was the 1962 "mistake" of a still-married man and a recently divorced woman, my husband was the unplanned baby of the family when his mom was 41 (not a good age to be pregnant back in 1961). Both of our adopted children are the result of unplanned pregnancies of young people in unmarried, uncommitted relationships! My whole family unit shouldn't exist, according to the criteria of needing to be planned and wanted. But here we are, by the grace of God.

My response:

Please tell me you are smiling right now! Isn't that story so incredible? What you don't know is that the family that's mentioned is a truly incredible family at our church, one that has shown so much love to our community, even at great personal cost. In fact, this email moved me so much that I decided to include snippets of her story as the conclusion to the series.

There's a member of our church who is wonderfully unfiltered, willing to tell me exactly what she thinks, feels, and believes. She texted me this message:

I wanted to thank you for talking on abortion. Over the years I've "come clean" to some of my life groups about my abortion. People get very hung up on the abortion and forget about the person so often. I do know that when I was 16, I made the horrific walk into a clinic, being yelled at and called names. If I had ever felt like I wasn't alone, I may have chosen differently. Christ died for this sin too. And through love I think we could change things. But I wasn't met with love, nor was I a Christian at the time. "Christians" hid in trees and stood in the driveway, yelling at me and telling me how horrible I was. Since becoming a Christian, I've had the honor to love and support young women, to try to help them cope and know they weren't alone. I don't know if any of them were ever considering an abortion, but I do know that if I had that, if someone had been there for me, shown me love, and made sure I knew I wasn't alone, maybe I would have done something different. I think some of the "worst" sins we commit come out of fear. Addressing this topic gives me hope that we can help women not be afraid, knowing they are not alone and understanding the love of our God because we show it through all our own broken pieces. Thank you.

My response:

I hope you and I can make things better the next time an unplanned pregnancy happens at our churches or among our circles of friends. As the following sermon will focus upon—"Abortion and the Church"—God has called us to meet the very real and very intense needs that many young women feel when they are drowning in worries and uncertainties as they consider their future as unprepared mothers. And, as this upcoming sermon proves, many people who get abortions are afraid and uncertain.

Most of all, however, I am grateful that the Holy Spirit has convinced this woman that "Christ died for this sin too," meaning that she is equally forgiven, equally loved, and absolutely welcome to worship Jesus with our church family.

A friend from social media reached out after the message:

I wanted to comment about your sermon on Sunday on abortion and the womb. I have to admit that early on I was concerned about the direction the sermon was headed, but I kept listening because I was drawn in. It was brilliant. The way you presented all of the different options for people made me think of an attorney addressing a jury and leading that jury to see the ONLY answer is at conception.

My response:

While I was grateful for the encouraging second half of this comment, what made me the happiest was the part about her concern for the direction of the sermon. It proved that one of my favorite ways to start a controversial subject was successful, at least in her case.

What is that tactic? To connect with the way that everyone in the room is feeling.

Flip back to the introduction of this book and read the second paragraph. What you'll find there is my attempt to let all kinds of different people know that I see them and know about their views of abortion. This isn't going to be a one-sided lecture from a guy who has never thought about, talked to, or immersed himself in the arguments from the other side. Instead, this sounds like someone who can summarize what I believe and why I believe it.

This two-sided kind of introduction has been a go-to in my sermon playbook. If you've ever read my book *Gay & God*, you might know that I took the same approach with the topic of sexuality. I deeply wanted everyone to know that, whatever they believed or however they behaved, I was glad they were in the room. Their views mattered enough to me that I had come to understand them the best that I could.

Too often I come up short of that desired goal, so this woman's feedback was a great encouragement to me as I thought about continuing the series the following Sunday.

One of the more interesting and powerful emails I received came from a woman who wrote:

There is a billboard, or at least there used to be, on the interstate. I would pass that billboard when my grandma drove the two of us back from trips to visit her siblings. Leaving to go on those trips made me the happiest a child in my circumstances could be, and coming back—passing that billboard—brought nothing but misery. The message was meant to be uplifting, but the effect on me was exactly the opposite. The message simply said, "Smile. Your mother was pro-life." What a slap in the face for a young child whose mother made sure that the child knew that the mother's life would have been better without the child.

That billboard has haunted me since I first read it at the ripe old age of seven? You see, many people think that life is the greatest gift a person can be given. How wonderful it would be if that were true. In reality, though, viewing life as a gift is a privilege.

While I genuinely believe that people are entitled to their own opinions and that we have no right to judge others for their opinions (after all, I think this email has revealed how little we know about those around us and what experiences shape their perspectives), I refuse to acknowledge pro-life as a valid stance. If you say you are pro-life, whose life are you for? In general, this argument is made in support of the babies, but what happens when carrying a baby to term jeopardizes a woman's life? Are we not then trading one life for another? If we make abortion illegal, we are not eliminating abortions; we are simply removing access to safe abortions. Are we then not risking multiple lives?

Many people who preach in favor of pro-life policies are not considering what happens to babies after they are born. A child born is not a child fed, housed, educated, or loved (this paraphrased quote belongs to a Catholic nun, I believe). No, these pro-lifers actually seem to be pro-birth. They want the babies born. But then what? Does our society support these babies, raise these babies, mentor, clothe, advocate for, cherish, or value them? Segments of our society pressure women into birthing babies but give no consideration to the circumstances that created the unwanted pregnancy in the first place or quality of the unwanted child's life both during pregnancy and after birth. Some of the mothers are drug addicts, alcoholics, or prostitutes. Some conceived the babies after being raped. Some are barely making ends meet as it is. Who protects these children? Does our society care about the children who are beaten, abused, starved, abandoned while the "mother" goes off in search of her next high? No, our society does not. Go ahead. Ask me how I know. What happens to these children, then, who grow up without proper nutrition, appropriate developmental stimulation, or a decent education? The cycle continues. The children might overcompensate by seeking out love and affection from anyone who offers it. They might fall so far behind in their studies that they drop out of school. They might numb their own pain by turning to a lifestyle filled with drugs and alcohol. Stereotypes are created, and society latches onto them and perpetually punishes the unwanted children who may then have unwanted children of their own.

Maybe more accurate terms would be pro-birth, anti-choice, or anti-abortion; but pro-life is not a valid argument.

Yet somehow Christians have turned into single-issue voters. They refuse to vote for a politician who does not 100 percent oppose abortion. Let us for a moment forget about the children, because these voters have already done that. Let's think about all of the other issues that Christians are then ignoring. Do voting rights matter? What about racism? immigrants? pollution? corruption? closing the pay gap? healthcare? crime? clean drinking water? What is it about forcing women to birth unwanted babies that is so important to these Christians, especially when our society scoffs at providing social welfare benefits that would allow parents to feed and house these babies that Christians are so adamant be born? These Christians— for the most part—are talking about things that they have not experienced and cannot possibly understand. They hate abortion so much that they demand funding be removed from clinics that provide free services and life-saving services like mammograms and cancer screenings to women who do not have health insurance, cannot afford to visit a doctor, and have nowhere else to go. Is that not also trading lives? They refuse to acknowledge the good, instead fixating on what they perceive to be the bad. It is really not surprising that our society has seen a complete breakdown of family units. Our society does not care about the baby, let alone the family. Our society simply wants to control it.

I will admit that I have not listened to the first sermon yet. My husband and I are intentionally a week behind be-cause our tiny dictator (as we lovingly call our daughter!) has turned our world upside down, and church no longer works for our family. I don't know if—or when—I will find the strength to listen to your message. I'm too afraid. Part of me is also taken aback at the timing of the message (it is impossible to ignore the current political climate; was the timing intentional or merely happenstance?).

When people hear my story (we have only touched the surface of it here), they have one of two reactions: 1) I should write a book; and/or 2) how did I survive? How am I a living, breathing, mostly functioning adult? I am the exception. I am stubborn and determined, and I refused to fail. But I am the exception. I barely made it out, and I am not without trauma and scars from it. I only make it *look easy. At the end of the day, no matter how we cut it, slice it, or dice it, we are talking about children who are not wanted. When human lives are not valued, there are no winners and there are no losers. There are only victims.*

My response:

When I read this heartfelt email, I had two reactions— I painfully winced, and I gratefully hoped.

I winced because of the details mentioned that hinted at a truly traumatic childhood. My heart recollected other women from our congregation who have told me about the unspeakable horrors done to them by the hands of sadistic parents, so I am aware of just how deep these wounds can reach. The raw words reminded me that the simplest assumptions ("I'm happy my mom kept me") might not be true for all. Some have not been blessed with loving parents. Many have not lived a life where they felt loved. In such cases, it is time to weep with those who weep and mourn with those who mourn, reminding them that **"the Lord is close to the brokenhearted and saves those who are crushed in spirit"** (Psalm 34:18).

I didn't just wince, however. I also hoped. I had already written the second sermon in this series, a message that attempted to address so many of the issues mentioned by the author of this email. To her point, many Christians are passionately pro-womb but barely lift a finger to prove they are pro-woman. That needs to change. I hope it changes.

If she finds the strength to listen to this message, I hope she finds that I, our church, and our God care immensely about both the womb and the woman.

Sermon 1 Reflections

Your thoughts . . .

1. Read and think about 1 John 1:8–10. How would you apply these words to the issue of abortion?

If we confess our sins, he is faithful and just and will forgive us our sins and purify us from all unrighteousness.

1 John 1:9

2. If everything in the universe was created by and, therefore, belongs to God, what questions should Christians ask that non-Christians might not consider when addressing an issue like abortion?

You created my inmost being; you knit me together in my mother's womb. Your eyes saw my unformed body.

Psalm 139:13,16

3. Evaluate: A good church should be a place where abortion is talked about openly.

Surely I was sinful at birth,
sinful from the time my mother conceived me.

Psalm 51:5

Your prayer . . .

Sermon 2
Abortion and the Church

We started a conversation about abortion, because abortion is an issue that eventually affects all of us. In a country where 1 in 4 women will have an abortion and many more will consider it, where many men are involved and parents and friends and churches, abortion is real and relevant and important for us to talk about. Last time we zoomed into the womb and asked, "When does life begin?" We looked at the five main answers to that question—conception, recognition, viability, desire, and birth—and then we opened our Bibles and learned that, according to God, life begins at conception. That makes abortion, unless it's required to save the mother's life, a sin. If abortion is part of your story, please remember that Jesus died on a cross for every sin so that we could come to him with even this and be forgiven, accepted, and saved.

And that's about all I knew as a teenager. If you would have asked a teenage me, the issue of abortion was black and white, short and sweet. During middle school, my church showed me these same passages and then showed me a video of what happens in a later term abortion. It was, as you can imagine, graphic. It was an argument from recognition. That looks like a baby. That is a baby. Just like the Bible says. So, everyone, don't get an abortion. For many years, that's about all I had learned about abortion.

But since then I have learned a lot more. Especially from having kids. My daughters are amazing, but raising them is hard. And expensive. And exhausting. (I do love you, girls, really.) And—get this—I have everything in my favor. I am married to a great, godly woman who teaches little kids for a living, for goodness sakes! We have two incomes, money in the bank, and tons of support from our safe and ready-to-help parents. There was no shame or embarrassment in our pregnancies, little to fear besides sleepless nights and blowout diapers. Yet, despite all of that, those kids challenge us and changed our lives.

So imagine when the situation is much more complicated, when you barely know each other, when there are red flags with the father, when birth will bind you together forever, when you're depressed or addicted or broke, when your parents are pushing for abortion, when you can't predict your church's reaction. There's a book that reminded me of that. This book is called *Shout Your Abortion*, and it's a collection of dozens of stories of women who got abortions and why. Most of you have experienced or at least heard of the heartbreaking cases of assault or incest, two reasons why we get why it would be so tempting to abort. To be fair, even Planned Parenthood admits that such cases are extremely rare—less than one half of one percent of abortions happen for these heartbreaking reasons—but there are reasons. And compassion requires Christians to consider those reasons, not just what happens during abortion but why abortion happens. Teenage me never went there mentally, never wrestled emotionally with how saying no to abortion means saying yes to an unplanned, complicated, completely changed life.

So, church, what can we do? As followers of Jesus, saved by his love, filled with his Spirit, on a mission to love God and love people, what should we do? Here's the answer I want to unpack with you today—*Be Pro (Every) Life*. Many Christians speak, post, and pray for life inside the womb. Today, God wants to encourage us not to care just about that life but about all the lives involved when someone is pregnant and didn't plan it.

Let's ground ourselves in this incredible description of the early Christian church: **"God's grace was so powerfully at work in them all that there were no needy persons among them. For from time to time those who owned land or houses sold them, brought the money from the sales and put it at the apostles' feet, and it was distributed to anyone who had need"** (Acts 4:33–35). There were no needy persons among them. The first Christians saw needs, and they met them. Even if the needs were great, even if the needy were many, they sold their homes, they sold their land to show their love. Because the early church was pro-life. Pro (every) life.

So connect that to an unplanned pregnancy. What are the needs that make abortion so tempting? What fears are people facing that we, as their church family, could ease? I can think of three major needs:

First, there are *spiritual needs*. For some, perhaps for many, the need is truth. Planned Parenthood tells us that the number-one and number-three reason women have abortions is convenience. "The timing isn't convenient. I got school or work. My kids are grown, and I don't want to do the infant thing again." It's not an abusive father or a personal addiction but a preferred life that they don't want to give up. In that case, we need truth. That's life within you, a life that God made, a life that God loves. It would be murder to end that life, a gross injustice, and God won't stand for it. You can't. You must not. You shall not murder.

For others, however, the spiritual need is not truth but love. Sex is a sin that sometimes "shows." Unlike 98.7 percent of sins, an unplanned pregnancy can't be covered up. And that can bring shame. When you're starting to show, you wonder what the church people will say, how they'll look, how they'll judge. Satan loves to make church people judgmental and loves to make single moms feel they're being judged even when they aren't. So you and I need love. Lots of love. Evident, obvious, impossible-to-miss love. Smiles. Hellos. Sit-next-to-me love. You-belong-here love. I'm-glad-you-came love. I'm-glad-you-both-came love. Jesus-forgives love, Jesus-welcomes love, Jesus-is-pro-me-and-you-by-grace love.

Earlier this year I met a man who worked for a pro-life ministry who, along with his wife, invited a young woman to stay in their guest bedroom while she got on her feet. But the girl liked to party and, one day, found herself pregnant. Since she knew they were church people and since she had grown up with a strict religious father, she assumed her sin meant she was no longer welcome in their home. "I'll leave," she mumbled to the husband abruptly one morning. But this man—thank God—saw her need and met it. He gave her grace. He spoke to her of Jesus' love. **"Where sin increased,"** Paul wrote, **"grace increased all the more"** (Romans 5:20). The husband met her spiritual needs. And we do too when we apply grace to those who need it most.

But the needs are more than just spiritual. Second, there are *financial needs*. According to a 2004 Planned Parenthood survey, 23 percent of abortions happen for financial reasons.[8] Giving birth isn't a bargain these days. Medical bills, then diapers, then formula, then decades of financial needs. The love of money might be a root of all kinds of evil, but the lack of money is a root of all kinds of reasons, reasons to get an abortion.

Which is where we come in. Would you sell your cabin to save a kid? Would you drive your car into the ground to convince them to keep their baby girl? Would you put off your retirement, skip a vacation, give before you've done these things for yourself? Would you budget for our church's Good Samaritan Fund so our leaders are ready to meet the financial needs within our church family? Would you personally say to a scared friend or a worried niece, "We got you. Whatever it costs, we got you"? Could we, like the early Christian church in Jerusalem, create a culture with no needy people, where no one has to starve or shiver or abort because they're broke? Jesus' brother James wrote, **"Religion that God our Father accepts as pure and faultless is this: to look after orphans and widows in their distress"** (James 1:27). In Jewish culture, orphans and widows had great needs and few resources. In our day, single moms are the same. God loves it, accepts it, smiles upon it when we look after those in need. So before this moment passes, before the marketers tell us all the things we still need, would you take a step, make a gift, meet a financial need?

Finally, there are *relational needs*. If she keeps the baby, she might need help. Moms, she might need to learn how to be a mom because this just happened, unplanned. Guys, that wide-eyed guy might need to learn how to step up, how to grow up, what men do when they put down the controller and pick up a box of wipes. They might need mentors, babysitters, counselors, us. Church, that child will need us to love and accept and affirm. If there's not a dad in the picture, that child will need some men to model the faith for him, to take him under their wing, to remind him who he is and *whose he is*. Or, if she chooses adoption (a great option!), she will need support, love, resources, or maybe you to step forward and open your own arms and home. Some will say that abortion is better than giving birth and handing your baby to another family, but that's not true. God loves adoption. Jesus himself was raised by a man who wasn't his biological father. Every Christian has been adopted into God's family (Romans 8:15), which is why so many Christians love and support adoption itself. Make no mistake, that kind of love is work. Sacrificial work. Costly work. But Christ-like work. Paul wrote, **"Therefore, as we have opportunity, let us do good to all people, especially to those who belong to the family of believers"** (Galatians 6:10). Let's do good. Let's meet needs.

Soon after the apostles died, the early church had to navigate life in the Roman world. The Romans, as you may have heard, did not love children. Not only did they abort them; they also exposed them. During the first days after birth, people just took their kids and left them outside to die. If they were sick or handicapped or the "wrong" gender, they exposed them to the elements, to the animals. But guess who showed up? The Christians. The Christians picked up the babies, adopted them, and raised them as their own. In fact, this was so common that churches quickly became the place where the pagans abandoned their infants. Leave those little lives with the church. They'll love them. They are pro (every) life.

You're pro (every) life because you know how much you are loved. You know how pro (every) life Jesus was. And is. And always will be. Think back two thousand years to whom and how and how much Jesus loved. The lives of lepers and adulterers and prostitutes and tax collectors. Jesus loved and, despite the messiness, didn't abort his mission, because he wanted you in his family. Yes, Jesus saw the surveys, knew all the reasons why we sinned, the powerful reasons and the pathetic ones, the ones that kind of made sense and the ones that were completely senseless, and yet—yet—what did Jesus do? He loved us all the way to eternal life. He met every spiritual need. When Jesus died on a cross and rose from the dead, he made a promise that, through faith in him, God would adopt us as his own children, that our Father would not abandon us as bastard sinners but that he would set the table with a place for us, that he would leave the light on and the door unlocked so we could always come home, always have a room to rest, always have grace to come back to. Jesus died to plant a cross in front of that door when we sheepishly said, "I'll leave now," refusing to let sin evict us from the arms of God. The sexually immoral and the selfish, the abortionist and the apathetic, all of us can come to Jesus and have every need met, every sin erased, every mistake covered so that God would be pro-life, pro-your-life, pro-eternal-life. Romans 10:11 promises, **"Anyone who believes in him will never be put to shame."** Anyone—that's you—who believes in him—that's Jesus—will never—never, ever, ever—be put to shame. We will always belong. Because Jesus was pro-you-and-God-together-forever life.

Call me a spiritual optimist, but I think that truth has changed you. Look around for a second. Look at this church, this screen, these stones, this stage. You gave so much to build a church. I think you'd do more for a child. You gave to help this ministry. I think you'd do more for a mom. Yes, it will be messier. This building looked neat and tidy after nine months, and raising a kid isn't like that. But I think you're willing to love everyone, to be pro (every) life.

Viewer Reactions to "Abortion and the Church"

A young mother from church responded:

> *Really great message tonight. . . . And I just have to share a recent photo of deep gratitude and blessing for my little*

son, who was recommended to be aborted. What a glorious Father we have!

My response:

Proverbs chapter 3 comes to mind: **"Trust in the LORD with all your heart and lean not on your own understanding"** (verse 5). The God who guides us with his Word knows more than all the friends, family, and doctors combined. Therefore, we put our trust in him and believe that, through healthy babies or sick ones, he is able to bless us in ways we could never anticipate or expect.

A passionate woman of God challenged me with a text:

Hope you're ready to step up because I just told a sad mama we will help her. She is a recovering heroin addict, has a six-month-old with a man who hurts her, and her dad is telling her she has to leave his home with her six-month-old if she doesn't abort.

My response:

Wait until you see what happens with this story. I promise I'll tell you before the end of this book, and I triple promise you that it is a story worth waiting for!

A short but beautiful email showed up in the church's inbox:

Do you know any Christian organizations in Appleton that support unplanned pregnancies? I would like to contribute. Or should I give to the Good Samaritan group at The CORE? Thank you!

My response:

Yes! I was hoping and praying that God's people would do more than just listen to my message, take a few notes, and go back to their lives. I was begging our Father that, motivated by the sacrificial love of Jesus, our church would love in selfless and evident ways. So thank you, Lord, for this fruit of faith!

The woman who shared the long story earlier in this book (the "26-year secret") followed up with her thoughts about this message:

I apologize in advance for another long email. There was only one thing that concerned me in your sermon. It was the point on the church sharing the truth. After reading your book Gay *and* God, *I felt you really understood how important it is to love the sinner before presenting the truth. With a crisis pregnancy, we don't have time on our side; however, it's still important to let the person know that we care about them first and have their best interests at heart. When you said that sharing the truth was the most important because the #1 & #3 reason for abortion is convenience . . . this is where I had to check myself. Examine my thinking to see if I'm just living in denial with my abortion clouding my judgment. Perhaps it is, and perhaps that's why it's important for me to share my opinion on this.*

But you know what I mostly, almost exclusively, encounter at the pregnancy resource center I currently volunteer at? Scared, hurting, broken women. Not one I have yet to meet would say "convenience" was the reason for contemplating abortion. Almost all of them are pressured by someone they love to have the abortion, some being threatened to be kicked out of their houses. Some threatened to have their current child taken away by its father. And those very rare exceptions? In our small, very rural community, three rapes resulting in pregnancy in two years (and yes, we coach them to hopefully come to the conclusion that two wrongs don't make a right).

This past Monday I coached a young woman who was told by her doctor that if she has another child, it would kill her. Leaving her two small children alone. Consider having to make that decision. I know, the minority, right? The minority that keeps showing up in my life for some reason.

Don't get me wrong, women in a crisis pregnancy do need to know the truth. They need to know it's a life created and dearly loved by God that they're pregnant with. However, they need to know they're just as dearly loved by him too. Just how many of those women are going to be reached if they feel judged that their major life crisis is just deemed a "convenience" choice by those in the church?

People in crisis make poor decisions. Especially when they are scared and alone. Especially when they're already broken. Please know that I really appreciate everything you have been preaching about in this series. I believe that it is obvious you care. I'm not trying to nitpick your sermon. I just wanted to bring your attention to how that statement came across to me and may have come across to other women and men who are affected by this issue . . . and Christians who don't need any more fuel to hate these women even more.

Thank you for listening.

My response:

I was actually on a three-day vacation when this email arrived, so I didn't have the chance to respond to it for a few days. Before I could get back to the office and type my reply, however, she emailed again:

Pastor Mike, I have wanted to take back that last email

since sending it. I appreciate you tackling this issue that so many have ignored from the pulpit. Instead of encouraging you on, I was that critic that you really didn't need. I'm sorry. I feel you have been your best at trying to balance all these hard points of view on a very difficult subject. Looking forward to following along tomorrow. Praying for the Holy Spirit to give you the words and for him to open my heart (and others) to whatever I need to hear on this subject.

My response:

I had to smile at the humility, kindness, and thoughtfulness of this woman. Just like any job, being a pastor comes with more than its share of criticism. Being a pastor who communicates through mass media, the feedback (both compliments and critiques) comes in massive amounts. So I was touched by this dear sister's desire to encourage me and build me up for the finale of the series.

However, I think her first email was spot-on, needed, and wise. And her analogy persuaded me. When I preached/wrote *Gay & God*, I intentionally tried to lead with love, to surprise people with my unwavering commitment to love the entire world (straight, gay, bisexual, etc.) as much as God loved it when he sent his one and only Son. In retrospect, that love opened doors to share truth in a fresh way.

This message lacked that. I rushed to truth too quickly, making the "convenience factor" my first example of my first point. Perhaps a few people in church that day needed the blunt reminder, but it is far more likely that many more people needed to hear God's grace first.

The reformer Martin Luther once said that a person who knows when to share the hard truths of God's law and when to share the good news of God's grace should receive a doctorate in theology. While those two key teachings are easy to list on paper, knowing when and how and in what order to say them is incredibly challenging.

So your point is received and taken to heart, sister. Thank you for the courage to say it, even if you took it back a few days later.

A new member to our congregation responded:

So powerful and what a challenge for us as pro-lifers. And as GOD would have it, I just sold my Illinois house this past week!! I will definitely be in prayer as to how GOD wants me to use those resources. I have already located a right to life organization in my area. Thank you for your boldness in preaching and always rooted in GOD's Word. GOD bless you.

My response:

God's timing (or GOD, as she rightfully spelled it!) is incredible, isn't it? How often do you talk in church about the disciples selling their homes the very week that someone in church sold their home? Sometimes I just look up to heaven and shake my head at the way our Father works things out.

A couple listening online responded:

After listening to your sermon on abortion and the three things that the Christian church can do—meet spiritual needs, financial needs, and relational needs—we did something. We sent a $1,000 check to the resource center here in [our community].

My response:

Boom! Point, pro (every) life!

Another couple from our church family emailed another pastor on our staff:

We just finished Pastor Mike's second sermon on abortion, and we couldn't help but feel the Lord's calling to us. [My wife] and I are both in agreement that we would love to open our home and our family to adopt a baby that might otherwise be destined for an abortion. I don't know what the church's outreach is in this regard, but we plan to spread the message to our network of family and friends—babies are welcome here! We have a lot of love to offer and would be honored to be a saving refuge. Not sure exactly where to go from here. Maybe a phone call would be beneficial?

My response:

Boom! Double points, pro (every) life! Plus, wait to see how this story fits in with the story of the young heroin addict with the unplanned pregnancy. Speaking of her, another message showed up that week . . .

Hello. I have a heavy heart tonight as we don't have much time with [the young woman I mentioned]. Please pray.

Her dad is taking her on Thursday for the abortion. The girl's mom and I have shared everything we can about God's love for that baby and for her. I've offered to let her live with me and even offered to adopt the baby, but she is too afraid of her dad disowning her as he said he would, and he has already written off two of his kids, so she has to choose between her dad and this baby that she doesn't want but knows she is taking a life that God created. The mother is heartbroken and angry, as any mother would be when her ex-husband murders her grandchild.

I'll be in touch tomorrow . . . but for tonight please pray and pray some more that God works in her heart. Thanks much and God bless.

My response:

I can't imagine. As a guy who grew up with a loving mother and supportive father, parents who later celebrated the birth of my own daughters, I can't imagine having to choose between my baby and my father. A "heavy heart" is an understatement for the way the church feels about people stuck in such situations.

But God wasn't done with this story yet . . .

The church member involved in this complicated situation vented:

On a scale of 1 (not at all) to 5 (wow, are you even a Christian?), how bad should I feel that at the moment I wish we still had the ability to call down fire and brimstone?

My response:

I'm glad we don't have that ability because we forget that God has the power to do more than any of us ever imagined. If you need proof, keep reading!

A day later she messaged:

It strikes awe in my heart every time God acts in big ways. The young woman I've told you about has ignored me for the past two days, but today she texted and said she did not go this morning [for the abortion]. That is a very good start.

And then came the best update of them all:

Literally, I'm stunned. Yesterday the father said to his ex-wife that there was no way she or her friend (meaning me) were going to stop this abortion from happening. He told her he had the power in this situation not her. The ex-wife's reply was, "I might not be able to, but God still can." He scoffed at her and said, "Yeah you and your God . . ."

It was that comment in addition to the whole forcing an abortion that made me have the desire to call on God to hit him with a ball of fire and brimstone. I felt bad about that, but get this. . . .When I talked to R. [the ex-wife] today, she had a story to tell me.

Last night, about the same time I sent that email to Pastor Mike asking him how bad is it that I want God to rain down some power on this guy and show him who has the real power, the dad was calling R. nonstop, and she was ignoring his calls because she was so upset and just praying nonstop. He finally texted her in all caps, "CALL ME NOW," and she thought, "What if our daughter hurt herself?" So she called him.

He said, "I don't know what just happened, but I think your God hit me in the head with a lightning bolt, and I think she should put the baby up for adoption. I don't understand this. It really was like a lightning bolt hit me in the head."

I'm glad it didn't kill him, but for real, that's not a coincidence. Is that not the most mind-blowing thing!? I really, really love our God!

My initial response:

(Me doing a happy dance and walking around fist-pumping in the air, shouting, "Yes!!!")

My further response:

Just wait. I'll tell you the rest of the story before the back cover. And, no, you cannot skip to the last page of this book to read it. God is teaching you the art of patience. First, you need to read the final message I preached in this series, which I believed would be the most challenging for the church people who heard it.

Sermon 2 Reflections

Your thoughts . . .

_Therefore, as we have opportunity, let us do good to all people,
especially to those who belong to the family of believers._

Galatians 6:10

1. Why is it common, even among Christians, to care more about the baby in the womb than about the other lives involved in an unplanned pregnancy?

2. Imagine if you yourself were pregnant and didn't plan it (or you had gotten a woman pregnant without planning it). What would be your top three needs? How might a local church that truly cared about you help you meet those needs?

3. Meditate on 2 Corinthians 5:14,15. How does the gospel of Jesus' love for us affect the way we treat our neighbors, including those who are facing an unplanned pregnancy?

Your prayer . . .

Abortion and the Government

While abortion has always happened, 1973 was a landmark year for the issue. A few years earlier, Norma McCorvey got pregnant and wanted an abortion. But she lived in Texas, where abortion was illegal except to save a mother's life. So under the name Jane Roe, she sued her local district attorney, Henry Wade. Eventually, the case made it to the Supreme Court—in a case titled *Roe v. Wade*—and abortion was declared by a 7-2 decision to be a constitutional right in the United States of America. In the years since 1973, Americans have debated that decision, defended that decision, voted to overturn or voted to uphold that decision. That's not news to you, is it? I bet that 99 percent of the conversations you've had or heard about abortion haven't been about your pregnancy or your friend's pregnancy but about all the pregnancies, about how Americans should think about all the wombs and all the women.

Some people have said every woman has reproductive rights and the government, which is currently about 75 percent *male* at the Senate and House level, has no right to invade her privacy, which would be an injustice. Others have said that abortion itself is the injustice, since it hurts an innocent person, a life that began at conception. Still others are in the middle, wanting abortion to be legal but rare, reserved only for the toughest situations like assault or incest. Some claim that if we go back to our old laws, people will go back to their old ways—seeking illegal, unsafe, "coat hanger/back alley" abortions. Others counter that such an argument totally ignores the person in the womb. Everyone looks at the total number of American abortions, which has decreased by about 50 percent in my lifetime . . . and everyone takes credit for the drop. Was it the conservative love for the womb that did it? Or was it the liberal love for women's health? Every election season, this issue often becomes the issue, with candidates stating their position and anxious Americans hoping for *their* outcome.

So what should a Christian think about that? If you trust in Jesus Christ. If the Bible is your ultimate source of authority, and if you live in a democracy where you can speak, post, march, and vote, what should you do? I think it's important to answer this question because in a recent survey, you, the members of this church, proved that you are all over the map on this issue, passionate about many different positions. While I wish the Bible just said, "Here's what 21st-century Christians should do with abortion legislation!" I haven't found that page . . . but I have found a few principles that guide us. Today I want to cover three main ideas that are essential for every American Christian to know—the biblical view of church and state, the application of that view to abortion, and the New Testament example.

So let's start with the biblical view of church and state. If someone asked you what God wanted the government to do, what would you tell them? It would be very tempting for followers of Jesus to say, "Jesus! The government should do what Jesus said, to enforce what Jesus taught. Vote your values, right?" Wrong. That wouldn't be true. That wouldn't even be biblical. This is not the Old Testament, the time when church and state were the same thing, a theocracy, when Moses was both the prophet and the president, the spiritual and political leader.

That's not how the New Testament church told us to think about the state. I've covered this in depth in a series called

Politically Incorrect, which you can find online (thecore922. com/), but here's the gist of the difference. The goal of the church is Jesus and preaching Jesus as Lord and Savior. But the goal of the state is justice, protecting the innocent and punishing the guilty. Your beliefs and actions, what you think and what you do, are the concern of the church. But the concern of the state is just what you do. Can you imagine if a cop said, "Miss, do you know how fast you were driving?"

"Um, the speed limit."

"True, but do you know how fast you wanted to drive?"

Can you imagine if a judge could use fines and jail time for not believing the right thing? If cops were arresting people for not being Christians? Um, no thank you. The church is based off the Bible; the state is based off human reason. The church relies on law and gospel, the dos and don'ts of God's commands and the done! of God's promises. The state relies on threats—if you don't slow down, pay your taxes, and obey, you will be punished. So, even for Christians, we should think of the church and the state as having different roles and different goals.

	Church	State
Goal	Jesus	Justice
Cares about	Beliefs and actions	Actions
Based on	The Bible	Human reason
Relies on	Law and Gospel	Threats

First Peter 2:13,14 says: **"Submit yourselves for the Lord's sake to every human authority: whether to the emperor, as the supreme authority, or to governors, who are sent by him to punish those who do wrong and to commend those who do right."** God sends government leaders—do you see it?—to punish those who do wrong and to praise those who do right. Punish the guilty. Protect the innocent. Justice. That's the goal of a good government. Justice, not Jesus.

Paul agrees with Peter: **"I urge, then, first of all, that petitions, prayers, intercession and thanksgiving be made for all people—for kings and all those in authority, that we may live peaceful and quiet lives in all godliness and holiness"** (1 Timothy 2:1,2). Why pray for the government? So we can live peaceful lives. So injustice doesn't rip us apart and leave us running for our lives. Why vote this way or that way? So the most people possible can live peaceful lives. Because the goal of the government is justice for all.

A few years ago, my daughters came with me to vote. They watched as I took the official form and exercised my constitutional right. They looked as I filled in the bubbles I thought were best. And then they leaned in as I wrote in my preferred person for office—Jesus Christ. Yeah, I did that once. Man, I wish I could vote for Jesus. I wish that he was an option, that he would rule with justice in everything he did. He would protect all the innocent people. He would punish all the guilty people. But—I'm not sure if you heard this yet—Jesus ain't on the ballot. Christians have to make choices. And what a Christian should do—a Christian who believes in the Bible's distinction between church and state—is *seek maximum justice.*

Which takes us to part two, the second thing I want to talk about today—How does that apply to abortion? We've talked about the issue of abortion in here, in the church, but what about out there, in society. Is abortion an injustice we should address with our voice and with our votes? Does abortion punish the innocent? Can we make the case, not with the Bible but with human reason, that there is an innocent person in the womb who has the right to be protected?

Hmm . . . how would you make the case that there is life in the womb? Like I did in my first message in this series, you might want to take an honest look at the scientific data. At the unique DNA that forms when sperm and egg unite. At the conclusions of medical textbooks on biology and the study of embryos. At the seemingly reasonable conclusion that a woman doesn't have 2 heads, 2 spines, 20 fingers, and 2 sets of DNA but, rather, that that woman is carrying another person. Or you might logically think through the common arguments for abortion and apply them consistently, as I attempted to do in my first message. Can we end a person's life because they can't survive without help? or because they're not fully developed? or because they have physical or genetic abnormalities? Do such arguments work with one-year-olds, or does the state call such acts an injustice? Or you could look at a picture from inside the womb. Just look. If you didn't have skin in this political game, if you were as new to this as a class of kindergarteners, what would you think of what you saw in the womb? No Bible; just reason. It seems, unless my bias for Jesus has blinded me, that it is reasonable to assume that there is life in the womb. And, if so, justice should protect that life from harm and danger, just like it should protect your life and mine.

"Okay, okay, Pastor. I need some time to think about all that. But are you saying that if abortion is also a justice issue, then every Christian should vote against abortion? Are you kind of telling me how to vote the next time I'm standing in the booth?"

My answer is no. I'm still telling you to seek . . . maximum justice.

Abortion is an issue of justice. If 862,320 innocent lives were ended by abortion in America in 2017, it's a huge issue of injustice. But abortion isn't the only issue that involves protecting the innocent and punishing the guilty. War is an issue of justice (many wars punish the innocent for land, power, and wealth). Race is an issue of justice (one of the grossest injustices in our American history). The way women are treated is an issue of justice (dismissed or undervalued because God gave them XX chromosomes?). Honesty and fairness and integrity and favoritism and nepotism and many other isms are issues of justice, and Christians who seek justice must care about all of them. I wish it were easier than that. Honestly, personally, I do. I wish Candidate A was perfectly just and Candidate B was perfectly unjust. Voting would be easy. But America isn't that. So we have to think. Brothers and sisters, we have to think. What policies are clearly, even on paper, unjust? What people have a history of supporting or avoiding justice? We have to learn as much as we can and then vote for someone who will do what God wants the government to do—to punish all the guilty, to protect all the innocent. And when someone asks us who we voted for, we can start with why: "I tried to seek maximum justice. And based on what I've seen and heard, I prayed and picked the person who would bring the most justice to the most people."

Whew. I told you this was the deep end. Now, before I say amen and give you time to wrestle with this teaching, I want to quickly cover one more part. What do we find in the New Testament? Jesus and Peter and Paul and James and John and Jude all lived under the authority of Rome, a non-Christian government that did not share their values. So if you could speed-read the books of the New Testament, what would you find? I think that's a fair question. The first century, from a church-state perspective, was much worse than 21st-centruy America, so what did that church do?

You would find a church that, on occasion, spoke up

against injustice out there but mostly preached Jesus in here. Yes, Jesus confronted the Roman governor with truth. Yes, Paul asked if his arrest was just, according to Roman law. It's there. But the focus is *in* the Bible. The Christians suffered under unjust governments but came home celebrating because they suffered for Jesus. The Christians weren't cowards—they would speak the truth—but they were most concerned with their calling. To preach Jesus. To change hearts. To use law and gospel, sin and salvation, truth and grace to get people to God. If today has challenged you, made you angry, made you question my theology, my only ask would be to read the New Testament and see what it says. Watch what they did. Witness what they said. Marvel at how they loved.

And remember what they believed about Jesus. That he forgives you. That he died on a cross to save you. That if you've gone all these years without thinking about this, without even considering that, if you realize you didn't support justice for all, look to Jesus. Jesus suffered under an unjust government so you could go free. When God's justice should have punished guilty people like us, Jesus stepped in, the just for the unjust, the innocent Lamb for those stained with sin, and he gave his life. Through Jesus, we have life— life as forgiven, accepted, good-enough-for-God-himself kind of people. Peter wrote, **"Christ also suffered once for sins, the righteous for the unrighteous, to bring you to God"** (1 Peter 3:18). There's no law out there that can offer us that, but there is a gospel in here that can.

Ten days ago I got an email from a member of our church whose family I greatly respect. Not only do they believe in Jesus; they have sacrificed so much to show Jesus' love to our community. They have dived into the deep end of difficult situations in order to love life, the complicated lives of those with addictions and abuse in their stories. But I never knew what that family had in common until she emailed me. She reflected on an American official who promoted abortion as a solution for unplanned, unwanted children and realized, "Our whole family would not exist if this was the case. I was the 'mistake' of a still-married man and a recently divorced woman, my husband the unplanned baby of the family when his mom was 14. Both of our adopted children are the result of unplanned pregnancies of young people in unmarried, uncommitted relationships! My whole family unit shouldn't exist, according to the criteria of needing to be planned and wanted. But here we are, by the grace of God."

I am so glad they are. Not just for the sake of justice but also for the name of Jesus.

Viewer Reactions to "Abortion and the Government"

After a lengthy post-church talk, she emailed:

This always happens to me. I think of what I actually wanted to ask later or how I wanted to say it. So is voting for the pro-life candidate just because you are pro-life wrong? I do look at other things, but that's how I usually end up voting based on that.

My response:

I can totally relate to this. Can you? I always think of the right things to say about 49 minutes after the conversation is over.

My short answer to this humble believer was, "No. Your rationale is not wrong. As long as you are not turning a blind eye to other issues of justice, being persuaded by the issue of abortion is not immoral.

What I was trying to avoid was a church culture that isn't concerned with issues of favoritism, bribery, racism, sexism, etc., simply because they stopped evaluating candidates after seeing their stance on abortion."

When it comes to God, we care about everything the Bible says (Matthew 28:19; 2 Timothy 3:16). When it comes to the government, we care about everything the candidate says. That's the only way to seek maximum justice.

A former couple from our church emailed:

Good morning from North Carolina!

First, we can't thank you and the pastors enough for the sermon series. We are blessed by your faithfulness, never compromising God's Word and not being ashamed to speak in love and truth the gospel of Jesus.

We both feel God leading us to reach out to you. If you know of any pregnant woman who needs support, spiritually or financially, please let us know. We are beyond honored to step up and let God lead our path. However that looks, we are ready, supporting her through pregnancy or being willing to adopt.

My response:

Thank you, Jesus. When I think about how life-changing and priority-shifting a child is, I am gratefully stunned by Christians who are willing to give up so much in order to show love. There is a maturity in faith in such people that I long to grow into, and emails like this call me to a level of love that stretches up toward the heart of Jesus.

Sermon 3 Reflections

Your thoughts . . .

1. Look once more at 1 Peter 2:13,14 and 1 Timothy 2:1,2. Based on what the passages say (and what they don't), how would you summarize the New Testament's goal for the government in your own words?

Submit yourselves for the Lord's sake to every human authority: whether to the emperor, as the supreme authority, or to governors, who are sent by him to punish those who do wrong and to commend those who do right.

1 Peter 2:13,14

2. Challenge: Study the platforms and positions of those running for election this year in light of the goal of the government to maximize justice. Then vote accordingly.

There is no authority except that which God has established. The authorities that exist have been established by God.

Romans 13:1

3. Read Psalm 20:7. Why is trusting in God the key to having no fear when it comes to elections?

Some trust in chariots and some in horses,
but we trust in the name of the Lord our God.

Psalm 20:7

Your prayer . . .

Christ also suffered once for sins, the righteous
for the unrighteous, to bring you to God.

1 Peter 3:18

Conclusion

And now, as promised, I want to tell you how all these sermons and all these responses combined to create one amazing opportunity for one young woman who found herself with an unplanned pregnancy.

Ready to read about it?

I have yet to meet the young woman from the emails I presented earlier. I only know that she is struggling with addiction, has a young child to care for, comes from a broken home, and is now pregnant.

On paper the details of her situation might cause me to lose hope. Except I know that God is working through his people.

God is working through the member of our church who has loved this young mother, counseled this young mother, opened her home to this young mother, and shared Jesus with her the entire time.

God is working through the two families who emailed our church to say, "If there is a baby that needs adopting, our arms and our hearts are open. Please let us know."

God is working through the sister in Christ who said, "I just sold my home, and I'm praying about how best to respond to your message."

God is working through the couple who opened their bank accounts and offered, "We are beyond honored to step up and let God lead our path. However that looks, we are ready."

God is working through the text I got from a staff member a few days after the final message was preached: "We just got a $7,000 gift to the Good Samaritan fund from a woman visiting The CORE who was moved by the abortion message."

God is working through the bold words of the girl's mother, words of truth that are filled with divine grace and "lightning bolt" power.

God is working in the heart of a man who once scoffed, "Yeah, you and your God . . ." and now says, "I think we should put the baby up for adoption."

As I type these words, the story is still in progress, messy and uncertain. But now our church family is ready and waiting, filled with grace and truth, aching to help and bless, no matter the cost.

If that is what happens in one church in one city in one state in one country, just imagine what could happen through all of us.

Through me.

Through you.

"And I pray that you, being rooted and established in love, may have power, together with all the Lord's holy people, to grasp how wide and long and high and deep is the love of Christ, and to know this love that surpasses knowledge—that you may be filled to the measure of all the fullness of God. Now to him who is able to do immeasurably more than all we ask or imagine, according to his power that is at work within us, to him be glory in the church and in Christ Jesus throughout all generations, for ever and ever! Amen" (Ephesians 3:17-21).

Notes

[1] *New Encyclopedia Britannica*, 15th ed., Vol. 14, "Pregnancy" (Chicago: Encyclopedia Britannica, 1974), 968.

[2] Dr. Willie Parker, *Life's Work: A Moral Argument for Choice* (New York: ATRIA Books, 2017), 12, 96.

[3] Amelia Bonow and Emily Nokes, editors, *Shout Your Abortion* (Oakland, CA: PM Press, 2018), 54.

[4] *Shout Your Abortion*, 77.

[5] *Shout Your Abortion*, 97.

[6] *Shout Your Abortion*, 88.

[7] Abby Johnson with Cindy Lambert, *Unplanned: The Dramatic True Story of a Former Planned Parenthood Leader's Eye-Opening Journey Across the Life Line* (Carol Stream, IL: Tyndale Momentum, 2014), 190.

[8] Luu D. Ireland, "Who Chooses Abortion? More Women Than You Might Think," *The Conversation* (July 27, 2018), https://theconversation.com/who-chooses-abortion-more-women-than-you-might-think-99982.

About the Writer

Pastor Mike Novotny has served God's people in full-time ministry since 2007 in Madison and, most recently, at The CORE in Appleton, Wisconsin. He also serves as the lead speaker for Time of Grace, where he shares the good news about Jesus through television, print, and online platforms. Mike loves seeing people grasp the depth of God's amazing grace and unstoppable mercy. His wife continues to love him (despite plenty of reasons not to), and his two daughters open his eyes to the love of God for every Christian. When not talking about Jesus or dating his wife/girls, Mike loves playing soccer, running, and reading.

About Time of Grace

Time of Grace is an independent, donor-funded ministry that connects people to God's grace—his love, glory, and power—so they realize the temporary things of life don't satisfy. What brings satisfaction is knowing that because Jesus lived, died, and rose for all of us, we have access to the eternal God—right now and forever.

To discover more, please visit timeofgrace.org or call 800.661.3311.

Help share God's message of grace!

Every gift you give helps Time of Grace reach people around the world with the good news of Jesus. Your generosity and prayer support take the gospel of grace to others through our ministry outreach and help them experience a satisfied life as they see God all around them.

Give today at timeofgrace.org/give or by calling 800.661.3311.

Thank you!